[A] Dialogue between a blind-man and death. By Mr. Richard Standfast ... Also, The great assize: or, Christ's certain and sudden appearance to judgment; ... By John Bunyan ...

Richard Standfast

[A] Dialogue between a blind-man and death. By Mr. Richard Standfast ... Also, The great assize: or, Christ's certain and sudden appearance to judgment; ... By John Bunyan ...
Standfast, Richard
ESTCID: T101786
Reproduction from British Library
Verse.
Edinburgh : printed and sold in Pearson's Close, 1735.
16p. ; 12°

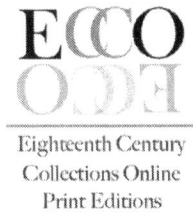

Eighteenth Century
Collections Online
Print Editions

Gale ECCO Print Editions

Relive history with *Eighteenth Century Collections Online*, now available in print for the independent historian and collector. This series includes the most significant English-language and foreign-language works printed in Great Britain during the eighteenth century, and is organized in seven different subject areas including literature and language; medicine, science, and technology; and religion and philosophy. The collection also includes thousands of important works from the Americas.

The eighteenth century has been called "The Age of Enlightenment." It was a period of rapid advance in print culture and publishing, in world exploration, and in the rapid growth of science and technology – all of which had a profound impact on the political and cultural landscape. At the end of the century the American Revolution, French Revolution and Industrial Revolution, perhaps three of the most significant events in modern history, set in motion developments that eventually dominated world political, economic, and social life.

In a groundbreaking effort, Gale initiated a revolution of its own: digitization of epic proportions to preserve these invaluable works in the largest online archive of its kind. Contributions from major world libraries constitute over 175,000 original printed works. Scanned images of the actual pages, rather than transcriptions, recreate the works ***as they first appeared.***

Now for the first time, these high-quality digital scans of original works are available via print-on-demand, making them readily accessible to libraries, students, independent scholars, and readers of all ages.

For our initial release we have created seven robust collections to form one the world's most comprehensive catalogs of 18th century works.

Initial Gale ECCO Print Editions collections include:

> ***History and Geography***
> Rich in titles on English life and social history, this collection spans the world as it was known to eighteenth-century historians and explorers. Titles include a wealth of travel accounts and diaries, histories of nations from throughout the world, and maps and charts of a world that was still being discovered. Students of the War of American Independence will find fascinating accounts from the British side of conflict.

Social Science
Delve into what it was like to live during the eighteenth century by reading the first-hand accounts of everyday people, including city dwellers and farmers, businessmen and bankers, artisans and merchants, artists and their patrons, politicians and their constituents. Original texts make the American, French, and Industrial revolutions vividly contemporary.

Medicine, Science and Technology
Medical theory and practice of the 1700s developed rapidly, as is evidenced by the extensive collection, which includes descriptions of diseases, their conditions, and treatments. Books on science and technology, agriculture, military technology, natural philosophy, even cookbooks, are all contained here.

Literature and Language
Western literary study flows out of eighteenth-century works by Alexander Pope, Daniel Defoe, Henry Fielding, Frances Burney, Denis Diderot, Johann Gottfried Herder, Johann Wolfgang von Goethe, and others. Experience the birth of the modern novel, or compare the development of language using dictionaries and grammar discourses.

Religion and Philosophy
The Age of Enlightenment profoundly enriched religious and philosophical understanding and continues to influence present-day thinking. Works collected here include masterpieces by David Hume, Immanuel Kant, and Jean-Jacques Rousseau, as well as religious sermons and moral debates on the issues of the day, such as the slave trade. The Age of Reason saw conflict between Protestantism and Catholicism transformed into one between faith and logic -- a debate that continues in the twenty-first century.

Law and Reference
This collection reveals the history of English common law and Empire law in a vastly changing world of British expansion. Dominating the legal field is the *Commentaries of the Law of England* by Sir William Blackstone, which first appeared in 1765. Reference works such as almanacs and catalogues continue to educate us by revealing the day-to-day workings of society.

Fine Arts
The eighteenth-century fascination with Greek and Roman antiquity followed the systematic excavation of the ruins at Pompeii and Herculaneum in southern Italy; and after 1750 a neoclassical style dominated all artistic fields. The titles here trace developments in mostly English-language works on painting, sculpture, architecture, music, theater, and other disciplines. Instructional works on musical instruments, catalogs of art objects, comic operas, and more are also included.

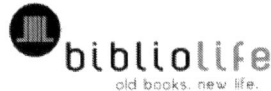

The BiblioLife Network

This project was made possible in part by the BiblioLife Network (BLN), a project aimed at addressing some of the huge challenges facing book preservationists around the world. The BLN includes libraries, library networks, archives, subject matter experts, online communities and library service providers. We believe every book ever published should be available as a high-quality print reproduction; printed on-demand anywhere in the world. This insures the ongoing accessibility of the content and helps generate sustainable revenue for the libraries and organizations that work to preserve these important materials.

The following book is in the "public domain" and represents an authentic reproduction of the text as printed by the original publisher. While we have attempted to accurately maintain the integrity of the original work, there are sometimes problems with the original work or the micro-film from which the books were digitized. This can result in minor errors in reproduction. Possible imperfections include missing and blurred pages, poor pictures, markings and other reproduction issues beyond our control. Because this work is culturally important, we have made it available as part of our commitment to protecting, preserving, and promoting the world's literature.

GUIDE TO FOLD-OUTS MAPS and OVERSIZED IMAGES

The book you are reading was digitized from microfilm captured over the past thirty to forty years. Years after the creation of the original microfilm, the book was converted to digital files and made available in an online database.

In an online database, page images do not need to conform to the size restrictions found in a printed book. When converting these images back into a printed bound book, the page sizes are standardized in ways that maintain the detail of the original. For large images, such as fold-out maps, the original page image is split into two or more pages

Guidelines used to determine how to split the page image follows:

- Some images are split vertically; large images require vertical and horizontal splits.
- For horizontal splits, the content is split left to right.
- For vertical splits, the content is split from top to bottom.
- For both vertical and horizontal splits, the image is processed from top left to bottom right.

DIALOGUE
BETWEEN
A Blind-Man and Death.

By Mr Richard Standfast *late Minister of Christ's Church, in the City of Bristol*

ALSO, THE

Great Assize.
OR
CHRIST's
certain and Sudden Appearance to
JUDGMENT;
or a serious Consideration upon the four last Things,
DEATH, JUDGMENT, HEAVEN, HELL.

By *John Bunyan* Author of the *Pilgrim's Progress*.

EDINBURGH,
Printed and sold in Peabody's Close, opposite to
the Cross, North Side of the Street, 1735.

DIALOGUE
BETWEEN
A Blind Man and Death.

By Mr Richard Standfast late Minister of Christ Church in the City of Bristol

ALSO THE
Great Assize:

CHRIST's
Certain and Sudden Appearance to
JUDGMENT,
With a Consideration of the Last Things,
DEATH, JUDGMENT, HEAVEN, HELL.

By John Bunyan, Author of the Pilgrim's Progress.

EDINBURGH
Printed and sold in Pearson's Closs, opposite to
the Cross, North Side of the Street, 1735.

Reader, perhaps thou'lt say, it is not fit,
These two Men's Works should make a Book com-
But why? If Moderation does attend (plete,
Thy Spirit, quickly all such Thoughts suspend.
In them's no Controversy, but each shows
Both bless'd Enjoyments, and eternal Woes.
They're dead, and reconcil'd with God above;
Read therefore humble Christians, read with Love.

A DIALOGUE BETWEEN A Blind-Man and Death.

Blind Man.

THE more Men see, the less they do enquire,
 The worse they see, the less they do desire
Others to grant what Blindness cannot give,
And for Intelligence grow inquisitive;
They ask to be inform'd, who cannot see,
I knew't by sad Experience, wo is me!

Death

Where are you, Sir? What sitting all alone?
I did suppose 'twas you by that sad Moan.
Coming this Way, to gather what's my due,
I thought it not amiss to call on you.

Blind-

I do not know that Voice, 'tis sure some Stranger,
And by his Words he seems to bode me danger.
    Death.
You guess aright, Sir, and before I go,
Know me you shall, whether you will or no.
   Blind Man.   (Name,
Why, what are you? Pray tell me what's your
And what's your Business, also whence you came?
    Death.
I will declare what no Man can deny,
There's none so great a Traveller as I;
Yet you must know I am no wand'ring Rover,
For my Dominions lie the World all over;
I march through Court and Country, Town & City,
I know not how to fear, or how to pity
The highest Cedar, and the lowest Flower,
Sooner or later do both feel my Power.
The mighty'st Emp'rors do submit to me,
Nor is the poorest tatter'd Beggar free.
In Peace I glean here one, and there another,
Sometimes I sweep away whole Streets together:
In Time of War, this much I can divine,
Whoever gets the Day, the Triumph's mine.
I am indeed a very great Commander;
'Twas I who conquer'd the great *Alexander*;
And after all the Victories he wan,
Compell'd him to confess himself a Man.
Were you *Goliah* great, or *Sampson* strong,
Were you as wise and rich as *Solomon*,
Were you as *Nestor* old, as Infant young,
Had you the fairest Cheeks, the sweetest Tongue;
Yet you must stoop; all this would nought avail,
For my Arrests will not admit of Bail.
For to deal plainly, Sir, my Name is *Death,*
And it's my Business to demand your Breath.
   Blind Man.
My Breath and Life shall both go out together.
          Death.

Death.
On the same Errand 'twas that I came hither,
I'll have both Breath and Life without Delay,
You must and shall dispatch; come, come away.
Blind Man. (Mind.
Why in such posting Haste? Pray change your
'Tis a poor Conquest to surprize the Blind.
Death.
You may not call it posting or Surprize,
For you had Warning when you lost your Eyes;
Nor could you hope your *House* should long be free,
When once your *Windows* were possest by me.
Blind Man
But Life is sweet, who would not if he might,
Have one long Day before he bids Good night;
O spare me yet a while, slight not my Tears!
Death
Hard Hearts and hungry Bellies have no Ears.
Blind Man.
I am not yet quite ready for the Table;
Death.
All's one to me, I am inexorable.
Blind Man
Nor by your Favour may I step aside?
Death
Be not deceived, 'tis in vain to hide;
My Forces are dispersed thro' all Places,
And I seize men without Respect of Faces.
I have a thousand Ways to shorten Life,
Besides a Rapier, Pistol, Sword or Knife;
A Fly, a Hair, a Splinter of a Thorn,
A little Scratch, the cutting of a Corn,
Have sometimes done my Bus'ness heretofore,
Be not so full that I need wish no more.
Should all these fail, enough of Humours lurk,
Within your Body, Sir, to do my Work.
Blind Man.
Yet then let some one run for my Physician,

A BLIND MAN and DEATH.

Tell him I want his Aid in this Condition.
Death
Run Boy and fetch him, call the whole College now,
For I intend to have them shortly too.
I value not their Potions nor their Pills,
Nor all the Cordials in the Doctors Bills:
When my Time's come, let them do what they can,
I'll have my due, so vain a Thing is Man
Should *Galen* and *Hippocrates* both join,
And *Paracelsus* with them too combine,
Let them all meet to countermine my Strength,
Yet they shall be my Pris'ners all at length.
I grant that Men of Learning, Worth and Art,
May have the better of me at the Start
But in long Running they'll give out and tire,
And quite the Field, and leave me my Desire.
As for those Quacks, who threaten to undo me,
They are my Friends, and speed some Patients to me.
Blind man.
Well, if I must, I will yield you the Day,
So 'tis enacted, and I must obey:
Henceforth I'll count myself among your Debtors,
For 'tis I see the Measure of my betters.
But tell me now, when did your Pow'r commence.
Death
My Pow'r began from *Adam*'s first Offence.
Blind Man
From *Adam*'s first Offence! O base Beginning,
Whose very first Original was Sinning
Death
My Rising did from *Adam*'s Fall begin,
And ever since my Strength and Sting from Sin.
Blind Ma
To know wherein the En'mies Strength doth lie,
In my Conceit is half the Victory
Have you Commission now for what you do.
Death
Yes, I Commission have, what's that to you.

Blind

A DIALOGUE between
Blind Man.
Yes, very much, for now I understand,
I am not altogether at your Command:
My Life's at his, who gave you this Commission,
To him I'll therefore go with my Petition;
I'll seek his Love, and on his Mercy trust,
And when my Sins are pardon'd do your worst.
Death.
That you may know how far my Pow'r extends,
I will divorce you from your dearest Friends;
You shall resign your Jewels, Money, Plate,
Your earthly Joys shall all be out of Date.
I will deprive you of your dainty Fare,
And strip you to the Skin, naked and bare;
Linnen or Woolen you shall have to wind you,
As for the rest, all must be left behind you.
Bound Hand and Foot, I'll bring you to my Den,
Where constant dreadful Darkness reigns, & then
Your only dwelling House shall be a Cave,
Your lodging Room a little narrow Grave;
A Chest your Closet, and a Sheet your Dress,
And your Companions Worms and Rottenness.
Blind Man
If this be all the Mischief you can do,
Your Harbingers deserve more dread than you,
Diseases are your Harbingers, I'm sure,
Many of which are grievous to endure;
But when once dead, I shall not then complain,
Of Cold or Hunger, Poverty or Pain.
Death.
There's one Thing more which I to Mind do call,
When once I come, then come I once for all;
And when my Stroke doth Soul and Body sever,
What's left undone, must be undone for ever.
Blind Man
That is a great Truth which I've learn'd to know,
There is no working in the Grave below,
To be before Hand therefore will I try.   That

A BLIND-MAN and DEATH.

That then I may have nought to do but die.
But tell me, Sir, do all Men die alike?

Death

To me they do, for whom God bids I strike;
Look how the Foolish die so die the Wise,
As do the Righteous, so the Sinner dies:
The greatest Difference will be hereafter,
But that's a Thing which is beyond my Charter;
That I to some prove better, to some worse,
To some a Blessing, and to some a Curse
That's none of mine, I dare not undertake it,
'Tis God's Appointment & Mens Works that make
Hence 'tis that Sinners Troubles never cease, (it,
But the End of the upright Man is Peace.

Blind Man.

There now remains but only one Thing more,
Will not your Power be one Day out of Door?

Death.

Must I needs tell you, Sir, 'tis certain true,
There is a Death for me as well as you;
And mine's the worst, for I must die for ever,
You may revive again, but I shall never.

Blind Man

By all that has been said, I plainly see,
You had no need t'ave been so rough with me.

Death.

Come let that pass, the kinder to appear,
I will reveal a Secret in your Ear:
The Death of Christ upon the painful Cross,
That seem'd to be my Gain, now proves my Loss.
All in his Hair the Strength of *Sampson* lay,
All with his Hair went *Sampson*'s Strength away.
I have no Strength, but what I had from Sin,
I have no Sting, but what lies hid therein;
Christ suffering Death to put this Sin away,
Hath made me his whom I suppos'd my Prey.
My Strength is now decayed, my Sting abated,
My Boldness check'd, and my Dominions stated.

And I am now both faint and feeble grown;
Much like to *Sampson* when his Hair was gone.
In my own Craft I was compleatly routed,
My Jaws were broken, and my Holders outed;
What now I catch, I have not Power to keep,
My very Name is changed from Death to Sleep:
'Tis true, I seiz'd on Christ, & brought him down,
And bound him in a Prison of my own;
But all my strongest Doors, Bars, Bolts and Bands,
Were but meer nothing in his mighty Hands;
He broke thro' all, and left the Doors wide ope,
And all his Servants Prisoners of Hope;
For tho' they die, yet with devout Affection,
They do express a joyful Resurrection;
And with their Master to be brought again,
That they with him may evermore remain.
Thus Christ by dying did become victorious,
And from his Bed of Darkness rose more glorious;
And I by binding him, made myself fast,
And his, I know, will prove my Death at last.

Blind Man

These Words give Comfort and Instruction too,
Henceforth I shall be better pleas'd with you.
Decreed it is for all Men once to die,
After that Judgment, then Eternity
To Prayer therefore will I join endeavour,
So to live here, that I may live for ever;
And seeing they that have and keep Christ's Words
Whether they live or die, be all the Lord's;
Repentance, Faith and new Obedience shall,
Fit and prepare me for my Funeral;
From whence I trust my Saviour will translate me,
In Season due, beyond their Reach that hate me,
Ev'n to that Place of Life and Glory too,
Where neither Death nor Sin hath ought to do
This Hope in me, that Word of his doth cherish
He that believes in me shall never perish.
Now welcome Death upon my Saviour's Score,

Who

A BLIND-MAN and DEATH.

Who would not die to live for ever more.

Death.

Sir, I perceive you speak not without Reason;
I'll leave you now and call some other Season.

Blind Man.

Call when you please, I will await that Call,
And while I stand, make ready for my Fall;
In the mean Time my constant Prayers shall be,
From sudden and from endless Death,
                Good Lord deliver me.

Judge not of Death by Sense, least you mistake it,
Death's neither Friend nor Foe, but as you make it;
Live as you should, you need not to complain,
For where to live is Christ, to die is Gain.

Mercy and Grace by Heavenly Pow'r
Can make the vilest Wretch on Earth,
  Forsake his Sins and Christ implore,
To Crown him with a second Birth

  So *Buynan* once lay wallowing in the Mire,
'Till Grace and Mercy set his Heart on Fire;
Drew him from hence with Bands or dying Love,
And crowned the Pilgrim's Head with Joys above.
Joys which a Thousand Deaths will recompence,
Joys which like God are lasting and immense.

THE

THE
Great Assize:
OR,
CHRIST's
Certain and Sudden Appearance to
JUDGMENT.

Job xiv. 2, 3.

Man that is born of a Woman, is of few Days and full of Trouble; he cometh forth like a Flower, and is cut down, he fleeth also like a Shadow, and continueth not.

O That poor earthly Mortals would attend
   With Seriousness of Mind to what is pen'd,
Here is presented clearly to the Eye,
A little World new made most gloriously
To Day here stands proud Man, like Flowers sprite
But look To morrow, and he is wither'd quite;
How happy might poor fallen Man have liv'd
For ever, had he not his Maker griev'd;

His

The GREAT ASSIZE.

His num'rous Off-spring never would espy,
Thro' that black Curtain of Mortality.
He might disdain Assaults, also defie
Grim Death; but now, alas! he's born to die.
Dust must to Dust, said God upon his Fall,
Entailing of that Sentence on us all:
Polluted nat'rally with that foul Sin,
Which did in *Adam* and poor *Eve* begin.
Alas! how swift the Days of Man pass by;
Swifter than Weaver's Shuttle do they fly:
As soon as Death doth end his Days, so soon
Man must appear before the great Tribune.
Death will no favour to a King afford,
Nor Difference make 'twixt Beggar and a Lord;
Beauty nor Riches, Favour will obtain,
He'll take no Bribes to mitigate their Pain,
Nor Florid Language can him satisfie,
For Death will tell him that he's born to die;
No Difference with Age and Youth he makes,
But each alike of Death participates.
You find *Methusalem* by Death was told,
That die he must though he was ne'er so old;
Like Fruit, when almost ripe, Storms can it shake,
So Youth when almost Man, Death may him take.
Search you Death's Lime Pits, and you'll find therein
As many young Steer, as the Oxes Skin.
Of all Things here, certain unto Man's Eye,
Nothing's more certain than he's born to die.

The Sinner trusting to Riches.
And yet how proud's a Man this Side the Grave,
As if he never should an Exit have!
Boasting, poor Worm, of an uncertain World,
His busie carping Thoughts with Care are hurl'd,
'Till wealthy grown, proud of his Bags of Treasure,
He trusts in Riches, taking all the Pleasure
His Heart can wish for; nay, he does controul

The Checks of Conscience to his precious Soul:
Says to himself, Soul take thine Ease, and spend
Thy Time in Mirth, ne'er think 'twill have an End.
Thus, thus the Sinner doth abuse his God,
And chooses Vice instead of Virtues Road.
He swears and damns, and imprecates God's Wrath,
To strike him dead; but ah! to Death he's loath.
He damns his very Soul, is it not just,
That God should do so too, and say, be curst.
Roaring and ranting is his hellish Note,
Quaffing so long, until his Senses float;
Drunk like a Beast, he staggers up and down,
Sleeps like a Hog, and is a Devil grown.
But Oh! if God thus anger'd, ready be
To say, thou Fool I do require of thee
Thy Soul this Night, come give a just Account,
To what thy Stewardship does now amount;
How dumb and senseless would he stand to see,
Hell ready to devour him presently:
Fruitless would be his Search to find a Place,
'Mong Rocks to hide him from God's angry Face.
For flinty Rocks, and Natures Hills that soar
Their tow'ring Heads so high, will be no more,
And all Things vanish by God's sov'reign Pow'r

※※※※※※※※※※※※※※※※※※※※※

Old Age with its Troubles
But now suppose God suffers him to live,
Adds Mercy unto Mercy, and does give
Him yet a longer Time of Life, and tries
If he'll repent before Death shuts his Eyes
He sees that Life runs round like to a Wheel,
And wrinkled Years upon his Brows do steal,
Besides gray Hairs upon his Head do grow,
Scatter'd it lies like to a Drift of Snow.
A foggy Dimness doth his Sight assail,

His

Sinking unto his Head his Eyes they fail;
His Tongue does faulter, and his Hands they shake,
And with the Palsie every Limb doth quake:
His stagg'ring Pillows cannot stand at all;
His House is so decay'd, 'tis near to fall:
His Age brings with it Sickness and Disease;
His Limbs so feeble are, seek sluggish Ease:
His Pleasure's gone, it doth him sore annoy,
To think of Youth's Delight and former Joy.
His Mind doth dream of Death before his Eyes,
And Death's pale Image doth his Soul surprize.

God's Mercy abus'd, Death sent.
His Glass just run, he's even out of Breath,
Ready to yield his Life to conquering Death,
Who will no longer favour his old Age,
But is resolved in his Death t'ingage,
It peeps behind the Curtain in his Face,
And draws the same, then dreadful is his Case;
His Tongue doth faulter, and his Veins they start
Like Sticks asunder, nay his very Heart
Ceaseth its Motion, and his Vitals gone;
So that at last he's colder than a Stone
His Kinsfolk dear his dying Eyes do shut,
And for his Bed into a Coffin put
But when his Soul hath parted clean away,
And left the Body like a Lump of Clay,
The Carcase is not colder than the Love,
Of Wife and Friends, who do forgetful prove.
And 'cause he cannot go he's carried forth,
Accompany'd by all his Friends of Worth.
Hir'd Mourners show his Years and Pomp so brave,
Convey him to his cold and sad like Grave;
But when they come to Death's pale Habitation,
And sees the Pit which gape with Desolation,
They

They throw the naked Coffin in, of all
His Friends, not one for Love will with him fall,
All get them gone, he still alone doth ly,
A rotten Worm bait, Tale of Mortality.

*** *** *** ***

The Vanity of his Wealth.
Thus ends his earthly Splendor and his Pleasure,
Wife, Children, Kinsfolk and his Bags of Treasure,
Are left behind to hold the same Estate
A little while, but follow must his Fate:
Nay, they're not sure t'enjoy it half a Day,
For Death doth oft sweep Families away
The Infant's instantly depriv'd of's Mother,
Husband from's Wife, the Sister from her Brother,
Children in Cradles often feel the smart,
Of conquering Death the King of Terrors Dart
Therefore, O Man, why art thou overjoy'd,
When all thou hast may quickly be destroy'd,
If any stormy Blast of Sickness blow,
All Features passeth like a Minute show.
Alas, poor Worm, what Thing canst thou call thine,
But sudden Death may quickly say, 'tis mine:
Behold thy Frailty! See thy Glass does run!
Therefore repent before the Time is gone
Both Young and Old have this before your Eye,
You're born to Happiness or Misery.
Think at Christ's coming, you must then arise,
And there be judged at the Great Assize.

Mathew xxiv. 41 *Watch therefore for you know
not what Hour the Lord doth come.*

***

The Manner of Christ's Coming.
Serene, like as the Days of *Noah* were,
So shall the Coming of our Lord appear. Eating

Eating and Drinking, they will merry make,
And carnal Souls Security will take;
Just like a Thief who cometh in the Night,
So will the Son of Man in Glory bright,
Come down with num'rous Angels, and the sound
Of Trumpets shril, un-nerving thus the Ground,
Ye dead arise; Lord, what a Horrour here
Is to the Wicked, who must straight appear,
And come to Judgment! O how this begins,
To bring to mind their many wretched Sins.
Conscience immediately appears, and must
Be the sad Soul's accusing Witness first;
Hanging their Heads, cannot endure the Shocks,
Of God's revenging Wrath; then to the Rocks
They run in vain, most miserable Elves,
To seek some shelt'ring Place to hide themselves.
Then are they separated as they stand,   Hind
The Goats i' th' left, the Sheep at Christ's right
O! the sad Skriechs they make, the rueful Cries,
To see Hell gaping just before their Eyes!
The Heavens melt away with fervent Heat,
The Earth is burning underneath our Feet:
The Books are opened, judged now they must,
Condemned next, then are pronounced curst.

The blessed Estate of the Godly.
But happy, ever happy are the Sheep
Of Christ, who Joy for evermore will reap,
When he shall say to's Saints, *Come, come ye thither,*
You of my chosen Flock, blest of my Father;
The Kingdom now enjoy, for you prepared,
Before the Word was made or Heavens rear'd.
O what Soul-ravishing sweet News is this!
Angels attend them presently to bliss,
With Glory crown'd, eternally they sing,
Hosannahs to their heavenly Lord and King.
Rivers of Joy before their Eyes run by,

Oceans

Oceans of Pleasure to Eternity,
Cloathed with Robes, shining like Jasper Stone,
They sing Christ's Praises on his heavenly Throne,
Angels attend these Saints, and what's more,
Joy hath no End, but lasts for evermore

The miserable State of the Wicked
But hark, what Grief the damned does attend,
Who have no Advocate to stand their Friend,
Sentence must passed be, *Go, go to dwell,*
In endless burning in the Lake of Hell;
Depart with Devils who did you entice
To hate your Saviour, and to cleave to Vice;
Go to that everlasting misery
Howling with foul Fiends perpetually.
O what a wretched Sight 'twill be to see,
The Devils dragging them to Misery!
Husbands to see their Wives convey'd to bliss,
Whilst they with damned Souls Salvation miss
Son from the Father, Father from the Son,
Must separated be i'th' Day of Doom
Praising of God, and own it to be just,
Their own Relations are with Devils curst
The Godly they to Heaven take their flight,
Whilst wicked take their Course to Hell outright

Lord let us watch continually and pray,
That we may be prepar'd for that great Day,
Give us Repentance that while here we live,
We may the Offers of his Grace receive;
And feed our Souls, O God, with thy free Grace
That we may stand before our Saviour's Face,
O grant that when the Force of Death we try,
We may cry out where is thy Victory?
And mounting up to thee, with Joy may sing,
Oh gloomy Grave where is thy bitter Sting?

F I N I S.

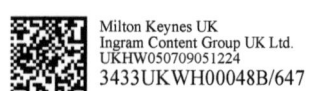
Milton Keynes UK
Ingram Content Group UK Ltd.
UKHW050709051224
3433UKWH00048B/647

An essay upon the nature and qualities of tea. ... By J. Ovington, ... The second edition with additions.

J. Ovington

An essay upon the nature and qualities of tea. ... By J. Ovington, ... The second edition with additions.
Ovington, J. (John)
ESTCID: T099425
Reproduction from British Library

London : printed for John Chantry, and sold by Ben. Bragg, 1705.
[6],40p. ; 8°

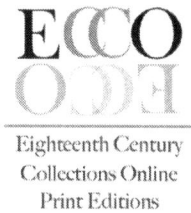

Eighteenth Century
Collections Online
Print Editions

Gale ECCO Print Editions

Relive history with *Eighteenth Century Collections Online*, now available in print for the independent historian and collector. This series includes the most significant English-language and foreign-language works printed in Great Britain during the eighteenth century, and is organized in seven different subject areas including literature and language; medicine, science, and technology; and religion and philosophy. The collection also includes thousands of important works from the Americas.

The eighteenth century has been called "The Age of Enlightenment." It was a period of rapid advance in print culture and publishing, in world exploration, and in the rapid growth of science and technology – all of which had a profound impact on the political and cultural landscape. At the end of the century the American Revolution, French Revolution and Industrial Revolution, perhaps three of the most significant events in modern history, set in motion developments that eventually dominated world political, economic, and social life.

In a groundbreaking effort, Gale initiated a revolution of its own: digitization of epic proportions to preserve these invaluable works in the largest online archive of its kind. Contributions from major world libraries constitute over 175,000 original printed works. Scanned images of the actual pages, rather than transcriptions, recreate the works ***as they first appeared.***

Now for the first time, these high-quality digital scans of original works are available via print-on-demand, making them readily accessible to libraries, students, independent scholars, and readers of all ages.

For our initial release we have created seven robust collections to form one the world's most comprehensive catalogs of 18th century works.

Initial Gale ECCO Print Editions collections include:

> ***History and Geography***
> Rich in titles on English life and social history, this collection spans the world as it was known to eighteenth-century historians and explorers. Titles include a wealth of travel accounts and diaries, histories of nations from throughout the world, and maps and charts of a world that was still being discovered. Students of the War of American Independence will find fascinating accounts from the British side of conflict.

Social Science
Delve into what it was like to live during the eighteenth century by reading the first-hand accounts of everyday people, including city dwellers and farmers, businessmen and bankers, artisans and merchants, artists and their patrons, politicians and their constituents. Original texts make the American, French, and Industrial revolutions vividly contemporary.

Medicine, Science and Technology
Medical theory and practice of the 1700s developed rapidly, as is evidenced by the extensive collection, which includes descriptions of diseases, their conditions, and treatments. Books on science and technology, agriculture, military technology, natural philosophy, even cookbooks, are all contained here.

Literature and Language
Western literary study flows out of eighteenth-century works by Alexander Pope, Daniel Defoe, Henry Fielding, Frances Burney, Denis Diderot, Johann Gottfried Herder, Johann Wolfgang von Goethe, and others. Experience the birth of the modern novel, or compare the development of language using dictionaries and grammar discourses.

Religion and Philosophy
The Age of Enlightenment profoundly enriched religious and philosophical understanding and continues to influence present-day thinking. Works collected here include masterpieces by David Hume, Immanuel Kant, and Jean-Jacques Rousseau, as well as religious sermons and moral debates on the issues of the day, such as the slave trade. The Age of Reason saw conflict between Protestantism and Catholicism transformed into one between faith and logic -- a debate that continues in the twenty-first century.

Law and Reference
This collection reveals the history of English common law and Empire law in a vastly changing world of British expansion. Dominating the legal field is the *Commentaries of the Law of England* by Sir William Blackstone, which first appeared in 1765. Reference works such as almanacs and catalogues continue to educate us by revealing the day-to-day workings of society.

Fine Arts
The eighteenth-century fascination with Greek and Roman antiquity followed the systematic excavation of the ruins at Pompeii and Herculaneum in southern Italy; and after 1750 a neoclassical style dominated all artistic fields. The titles here trace developments in mostly English-language works on painting, sculpture, architecture, music, theater, and other disciplines. Instructional works on musical instruments, catalogs of art objects, comic operas, and more are also included.

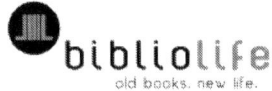

The BiblioLife Network

This project was made possible in part by the BiblioLife Network (BLN), a project aimed at addressing some of the huge challenges facing book preservationists around the world. The BLN includes libraries, library networks, archives, subject matter experts, online communities and library service providers. We believe every book ever published should be available as a high-quality print reproduction; printed on-demand anywhere in the world. This insures the ongoing accessibility of the content and helps generate sustainable revenue for the libraries and organizations that work to preserve these important materials.

The following book is in the "public domain" and represents an authentic reproduction of the text as printed by the original publisher. While we have attempted to accurately maintain the integrity of the original work, there are sometimes problems with the original work or the micro-film from which the books were digitized. This can result in minor errors in reproduction. Possible imperfections include missing and blurred pages, poor pictures, markings and other reproduction issues beyond our control. Because this work is culturally important, we have made it available as part of our commitment to protecting, preserving, and promoting the world's literature.

GUIDE TO FOLD-OUTS MAPS and OVERSIZED IMAGES

The book you are reading was digitized from microfilm captured over the past thirty to forty years. Years after the creation of the original microfilm, the book was converted to digital files and made available in an online database.

In an online database, page images do not need to conform to the size restrictions found in a printed book. When converting these images back into a printed bound book, the page sizes are standardized in ways that maintain the detail of the original. For large images, such as fold-out maps, the original page image is split into two or more pages

Guidelines used to determine how to split the page image follows:

• Some images are split vertically; large images require vertical and horizontal splits.
• For horizontal splits, the content is split left to right.
• For vertical splits, the content is split from top to bottom.
• For both vertical and horizontal splits, the image is processed from top left to bottom right.

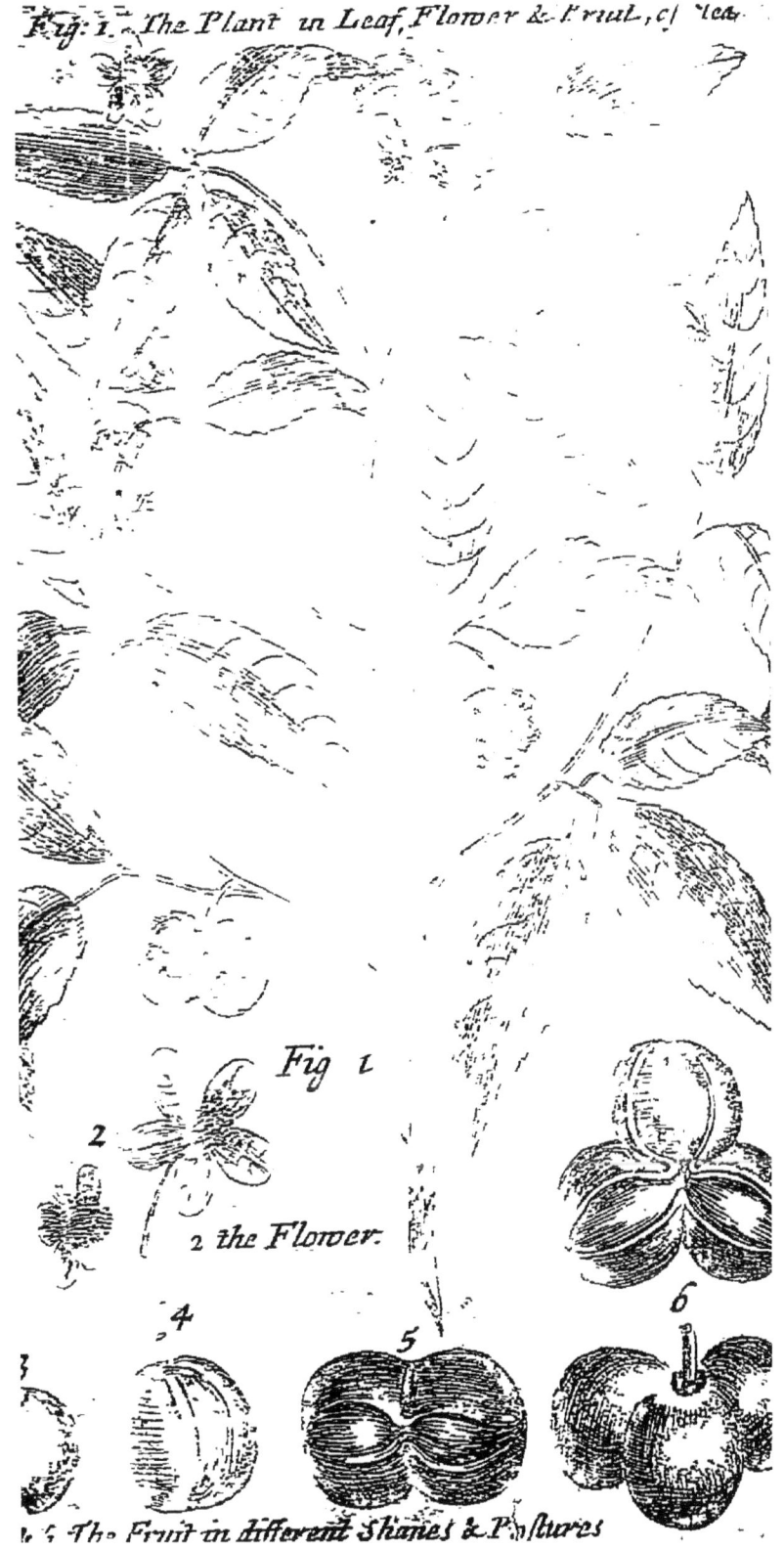

Fig: 1. The Plant in Leaf, Flower & Fruit, of Tea

Fig 1
2 2 the Flower.
3 4 5 6 The Fruit in different Shapes & Postures

AN ESSAY UPON THE Nature and Qualities OF TEA.

Wherein are shown,
I. The Soil and Climate where it grows.
II. The various Kinds of it
III. The Rules for Chusing what is best.
IV. The Means of Preserving it
V. The several Vertues for which it is fam'd.

By J. OVINGTON, D D Chaplain to Her MAJESTY

The Second Edition with Additions

THEA est de Cœlo missa terræ progenies,
Divini nominis æmula herba.

Pecini de usu Theæ

London Printed for *John Chantry*, without Temple-Bar, and sold by *Ben Bragg*, at the Blue Ball in *Avemary-Lane*. 1705 Price 6d

TO
The Right Honourable
THE
Countess of GRANTHAM.

MADAM

'TIS from your innate Goodness only, and that condescending Temper which is so remarkable in You, that this Foreign [Leaf] dares presume to Court Your [Favour], and hope for a welcome Entertainment. For where can a Stranger, that was always bred among a People the most polite of any in the World, expect a kind Reception with more Assurance, than from a Person, whose conversation is adorn'd with all that Civility that even China it self can boast of. And therefore while it [gains] Your Countenance, 'twill find [itself] as happy here, as if it still had stay'd at home, nay, rather with

Ad-

The Dedication.

Advantage to have chang'd its delightful native Soil, while it is under the more pleasant Influences of Your Protection.

But though the name of a Person, Madam, so Eminent as you are both upon the Account of Your Illustrious ORMOND Family, and those particular Accomplishments which give you so distinguishing a Character, were enough to recommend this healthful Herb to all that were in the least acquainted with the use of them; yet it is not it self destitute of some peculiar Virtues, which may justly claim a very favourable Encouragement from us.

For it is generally acknowledg'd to be both Pleasant and Medicinal at once, to delight the Palate and correct the Disease, and to heal the Distemper without giving any Disturbance to the Stomach.

The Dedication.

And certainly were the Custom of drinking it as Universal here, as it is in the Eastern Countries, we should quickly find that Men might be chearful with Sobriety, and witty without the Danger of losing their Senses; and that they might even double the Days of their natural Life, by converting it all into Enjoyment, exempt from several painful and accute Diseases, occasion'd very often by a pernicious Excess of inflaming Liquors, which render it rather a Burthen, than a Blessing to us.

But in pity, Madam, to this tender Leaf, I must cease from Panegyrick, least it should create a Satyr, and the innocent Praises of it be eccho'd back in sharp Invectives: For since its Constitution is so nice and delicate, as to be injur'd even by common Air, it will never be able to withstand the Malignity of an envious Breath, unless your Honour

and

The Dedication.

and Goodness interpose, which are so conspicuous, that Malice it self would blush to fix an Imputation upon them.

And from these Excellencies of Yours, which are the Crown and Ornament of Nobility, the Author hopes to find Your Pardon in the present Dedication, and that the Greatness of Your Mind will at this time show it self in Your Indulgence to,

Madam,

    Your most Humble and Obedient Servant,

        J. Ovington.

AN ESSAY UPON THE Nature and Qualities OF TEA.

Though the Use of *Tea* has for many Years past been highly approved of in the Empires of *China* and *Japan*, which are at present the chief Kingdoms that Cherish

An ESSAY upon the

with this *Celebrated Leaf*; yet since the *Europeans* by their frequent Navigations have opened a freer Trade and Commerce to those Parts, and have thereby been better acquainted with the Genius of those People, and their Manner of Life, they have thereby taken occasion to inform us, among other things, with the singular Esteem which those *Eastern Nations* harbour for it and of what daily Use it is among them. Whereupon this *Western World* has been induced of late to encourage the Importation of it, and make some Experiments of its admirable Effects, either out of *Curiosity*, because of its *Novelty*; or out of *Pleasure* of gratifying the *Palate*; or because of some *Medicinal Vertues*, with which it is pregnant. And since the Drinking of it has of late obtain'd here so universally, as to be

Nature and Qualities of TEA.

affected both by the *Scholar* and the *Tradesman*, to become both a private *Regale* at *Court*, and to be made use of in places of *publick Entertainment*, which has greatly rais'd the Character, and gain'd it a singular Repute; it might not be amiss therefore to draw up a short Account of its *Nature* and *Qualities*, to satisfy such as are its curious Admirers with the Knowledge of its Use. I will here discourse therefore of the *Climate* and *Soil* this Herb grows in, and its *various Kinds*; of the *Method of Chusing* what is best, and the *means of preserving* it; and the several *Virtues* for which it is fam'd. With an Answer to one Objection or two which are sometimes urg'd against it.

That which in *England* is called *Tea*, is in some other places pronounc'd

The Name of it

nounc'd *Tree*, especially in the Province of *Fokien*, which lies in *China* between 25 and 30 deg of Latitude. But there, they say the word is corrupted; for such as pretend to the genuine and primitive pronunciation of it, will have it term'd, according to the *Mandarin* Language, *Tcha*, and some *Tsia*. But how different soever the Name of it may be, the thing it self is universally agreed in.

The Mandarins are the great Men in China.

The Tree of Tea describ'd.

This *Tea* is a Leaf which grows upon a *Shrub* in *China* and *Japan*, not exceeding either in Height or Breadth our *Rose* or *Gooseberry Bushes* in *Europe*. The branches of which, from the Root to the Top, are cloath'd with abundance of tender Leaves of different Magnitude, though of the same Form and Shape. For *Coronius*, who liv'd several Years *ature and Qualities of* T E A. 5

the Empire of *Japan*, assures
That *upon the same Tree are
...ves of five different Proportions,
...largest of which resemble our Gar-
... Balm, and grow towards the
...ot; and as they rise in Height,
...ir Size decreases, but the smallest
...r the largest Price. The Seed
...it is round and black, which in
...ree Jews time after it is sown,
...duces new Plants. But the Flow-
... of it, which are all white, are
... Esteem the main Virtue is
...id in the Leaves When the
...vers however are new and
...sh, they yield a very pleasant
...ell; but in time as I have seen
...em, they grow yellow; and
...ing put into Water, turn it
...own. They consist of five
...itish or palish Leaves, with ma-
... Chives in the middle of the
...ower.

The

The Shrub it self is of a strong and hardy Constitution, is proof against Storms, and receives no Damage by Snow or Hail, and lives and thrives in those very Climates, the sharpness of whose Air might seem pernicious, if not fatal to its tender Leaf; for the Winter in *England*, in some places where it grows, is no more cold. The *stony Soils* are apt in *China* to produce the choicest *Tea*, though for the most part it is planted there in the Valleys and in light Ground. And might it therefore be convenient to have it brought thither, there is nothing in the Nature either of our Ground or Air that seem to contradict it's Increase among us. Especially if sufficient Care were taken for the safe and cautious Transportation of the Seed or Branches, and in their Growth they were expos'd, with the best
Advan-

Nature and Qualities of TEA. 7

[ad]vantage to the Sun. Though [th]e Art here used for raising of it [h]as not yet answer'd Expectation. [B]ut whether this proceeds from [th]e *Envy* of the *Chinese*, who are [sa]id to boil the Seed, lest it should [b]e planted any where else; or [fr]om the Age of it, or untimely [C]ollection of it, or the immode[r]ate Heat of the Sun, and variety [o]f Weathers in a long Voyage, it's [u]ncertain.

The *Spring* is reputed the most [p]roper Season for gathering the [L]eaves, because 'tis this time on[l]y of the Year that renders them [m]ost soft and delicate, juicy and [t]ender, which gives the Water [w]herein they are infus'd both a more pleasant Flavor to gratify the [S]mell, and a Taste more agree[a]ble to the *Palate*. And certain[l]y 'tis none of the meanest Signs of

The Season for Gathering it

8 *An ESSAY upon the*

of the remarkable Ingenuity
th_ *Chinese*, to prepare the *Lea*
with so much Art to make the
still continue *green*, notwithstand
ing all the Length of Time the
have been dried. Which I think
is not very usual with our drie
Herbs in *Europe*.

The several sorts of *te*

A Catte of about 20 ounces

A Mandarin is a Great Man in China

In *China* are several sorts
Tea, which are unknown to
in *Europe*, some of which are ve
ry cheap, but others are so high
ly valuable and much esteem'd
that a single *Catte* is look'd upo
as a present fit for a *Mandarin*
For so vastly different is the price
that one single Pound of that *Tea*
which is cultivated for the Em
peror, for the Nobility, and Lord
of the Court, is sold for more than
one hundred times as much as
another sort. And in *Japan*, tha
which is prepar'd for the Gran
dee

Nature and Qualities of TEA. 9

...es there, is both planted in the ...ost refin'd Earth, and carefully ...fended from all Injuries of the ...ir, from all exceſſive Colds and ...eats, and every thing that may ...apt to offend the tender Leaf. ...nd as at home they commonly ...ect the Entertainment of a nu- ...erous Multitude of Servants, ...d a ſtately Furniture of Inſtru- ...ents for the Preparation of their ...in the greateſt Magnificence ...d Splendor; ſo they want not ...road ſuch as are purpoſely im- ...oy'd to husband it with the ut- ...oſt Care and Diligence, as well ...with a peculiar Art. But that ...hich is generally brought into ...rope, is known only by theſe ...ree diſtinct Names.

'The three ſorts of Tea com- *Philoſoph*
...monly carried to *England*, are all *Tranſact for*
...rom the ſame Plant, only the July and Au-
...eaſon of the Year, and the Soil guſt. 1702. p.
     ' makes 1205

'makes the difference. The B[o]
'or Voui, so called of some Mou[n]
'tains in the Province of Fokie[n]
'where it is chiefly made, is t[he]
'very first Bud gather'd in the b[e]
'ginning of March, and dried [in]
'the shade. The Bing Tea is t[he]
'second Growth in April; a[nd]
'Singlo, the last in May and Ju[ne]
'both dried a little in Atches, or Pa[ns]
'over the Fire. The Tea-Shr[ub]
'being an ever Green, is in Flow[er]
'from October to January, and t[he]
'Seed is ripe in September and O[ct]
'ober following; so that one m[ay]
'gather both Flowers and Seed[s at]
'the same time. But for one fr[uit]
'and full Seed there are an hundr[ed]
'naught. Its Seed Vessels are [usu]
'ally tricapsular, each capsula co[n]
'taining one Nut or Seed. A[nd]
'altho' only two or three cap[su]
'la come to Perfection, yet t[he]
'Vestiges of the rest may be [di]
'scern'd. It grows in a dry G[ra]
ve[l]

Nature and Qualities of TEA. 11

...velly Soil, on the sides of Hills
in several places without any
Cultivation.

The first sort is *Bohe*, or, as
the *Chinese* have it, *Voui*, which
is a *little Leaf inclining to black*,
and generally tinges the Water
brown, or of a reddish Colour.
Those in *China* that are *sick* or
are very careful of preserving their
health, if they are weak, confine
themselves only to this kind of
Tea, to which they are willing
to ascribe a peculiar Virtue both
for *healing* and *preventing* a Disease, and extol it as a mighty
friend to Nature when it is
grown faint and languishing.
The taste of it when it is very
true and genuine, is delicious and
pleasant, and the weakest Stomach is able to bear it. This
kind of *Tea* therefore is both in
Colour and in Nature different

Bohe

This kind of Tea is of a healing Quality.

B from

from the other two, and ve[ry]
useful to such as are *wasting* a[nd]
consumptive, and excels the othe[r]
in its healing balsamick Qualit[y,]
and particularly in improving b[y]
Length of Time, which is ve[ry]
pernicious to the rest, for it gene[-]
rally grows better the longer it [is]
kept.

Singlo. The second sort is *Singlo*, [or]
Soumlo with the *Chinese*; [of]
which there are several kind[s]
according to the place of *Growt*[h,]
the manner of *preparing* it, an[d]
the *Nature* of the *Tea*. But th[at]
which is imported hither is [of]
two sorts, both equally goo[d.]
One of them is a *narrow and lo*[ng]
Leaf. The other *smaller*, and [of]
a *Blewish green Colour*, which tast[es]
very crisp when it is chaw'd, an[d]
afterwards looks Green upon th[e]
Hand, and infuses a pale Green[-]
ness into the Water. The Flavo[ur]

Nature and Qualities of TEA.

of it is fresh and fine, lively and pleasant. 'Tis strong and will endure the Change of Water three or four times. This *Tea* is brought over in round Totaneg *Canisters*, pasted over with Paper, and inclos'd in a wooden Tub, containing the Quantity of half a *Pecul* And that you may more plainly discern whether all of it be new or no, these two things may be observ'd. *First*, Examine the Leaves to see whether all or not of them are Green, if not, but that some of them are turn'd brown, or look *decay'd*, then may you guess that the *Tea* is not the finest, but is growing old, and will impair in Virtue daily. *Secondly*, Let the Liquor, into which the *Tea* has been infus'd, stand in a Cup for the space of a whole Night; if after this you perceive that it still continues green, the Goodness of it seems

Totaneg is a sort of metal brought from China. A Canister contains between 50 and 70 l. A Pecul is 132 l.

Means to know the best Tea.

unquestionable; but as it abates of this Colour, so, you may conclude, it has abated of it Perfection, and wants something of its Excellence and Strength. For the *fragrant Smell*, the *Green Colour*, and the *bitterish sweet Taste* are the distinguishing Characters of the Goodness of this kind of Tea.

The third sort is *Bing*, or *Imperial Tea*, according to the Epithet given it by the *English*; and by the *Dutch, Keisar*. This is a *large loose Leaf*, and therefore takes up more Room, proportionable to the weight of it, than any other *Tea*, because it is more open and spungy. The finest Sort of it looks both Green to the Eye, and is crisp in the Mouth, and the Smell of it is very pleasant, which inhances the Price of it here in *England*; and 'tis high-

highly esteemed likewise in *China*, being sold there at three times the Price of the other two. But it generally is of divers Colours, as Yellow, Green, &c. and is reputed Weak, spending it self quickly in the Infusion, and only tinctures the Water with any Spirit twice, because it is not put in weight for weight with other Tea. This likewise, as the others, is Imported in large thick Totaneg *Canisters* included in wooden Tubs, or in Baskets made of small Bam*boe* Canes.

These are those several forts of *Tea*, to some one of which all that is transported hither is commonly reduc'd; and in describing its Variety, and the different Properties of each of them, some Directions have been given for distinguishing what is choice and good, from what is mean and refuse, which Instruction I shall pursue with one Remark more, a little further.

'Tis necessary for all such as travel to *China*, nicely to understand the Nature of the Goods there, if they intend to escape the Cheats and Frauds, and to trade therein with Advantage. For such is the subtilty of the *Chinese* in their *Trade*, and so artificial are they in their *Traffick*, and so mightily intent upon their *Gain*, that they falsify every thing they sell, if 'tis capable of *Sophistication*, and he must be very quick and expert indeed, that has wit enough to escape in all things their Impositions. This they formerly practic'd even in their Sale of *Tea*, though the Advantage of it was inconsiderable. For with it they sometimes mixt some other Herbs of less Value, to swell the

…e Parcel and increase the Gain,
…d with this artificial Mixture
…ey cunningly dispos'd of it.
…ut the Prudence and Caution of
…e *Europeans* prevent at present
…l the fraudulent Attempts of
…is Nature. And yet such is
…e peculiar Talent of the *Chinese*
… the management of this Art,
…at the Discovery of them in
…e Trick, is only the quicken-
…g their Invention of another;
…d he that has thought himself
…fe in timely preventing of a
…all Cheat, has found after-
…ards how Weak he was, when
… his means he only tempt-
… them to over-wit him in a
…eater. And though 'tis pos-
…le to fix their Honesty for
…me time in that particular
…herein the fraud has been found
…t, yet will their inherent Pra-
…y soon exert it self in some-
…ng else, and make them kna-
vish

vish by Transmutation. Which occasions the wary *English* and *Dutch* Merchants in their Trading for *Tea*, to open many times both the *Top*, the *Middle*, and the *Bottom* of the *Canisters*, to prevent the Cheat of courser *Tea* which has been sometimes privately put into one place, sometimes into another.

The Method of preparing Tea. The Method the *Chinese* use in preparing of *Tea*, to make it dry and crisp, is, as some affirm, to put it in Ovens, or in Kilns, or to expose it to the Sun; or as others say, by frying it twice or oftner in a Pan; and as often as it is taken off the Fire, it is rolled with the Hand upon a Table till it curls. By this means the Leaves contract such a *Dryness* and *Hardness*, as inables them to retain their Virtue for many Years.

Though

ture and Qualities of TEA.

Though the Tree of *Tea* is for[m]ed by Nature against rigid [co]lds, against Storms and bad [w]eather, and is able to subsist and [no]urish even upon stony Ground; [bu]t the *Leaf* of it, when once [it] is prepar'd for Use, is of a [te]mper quite different; 'tis *deli[c]ate* and *tender*, injur'd by the [br]eath, and damag'd by the very [com]mon *Air*. And therefore the [Chi]nese knowing how subject it [is] to Decay, and how easily 'tis [tai]nted, carefully provide against [the]se Dangers, by keeping of it [ve]ry close, and at a Distance [fro]m all *strong smells*, whether [th]ey be *pleasant Flavors*, or *fœted [Sc]ents*. for both of these are [eq]ually pernicious, and destru[ct]ive of the natural Smell. And [tho]se that would secure it from [su]ch Disasters, must see that it [be] guarded from those Enemies, [m]ust look that it be kept from
any

Rules for preserving it.

Tottanege [?] *of Metal brought from China.*

any strong Odor that wou'd affect it, and shut it up securely from the *Ambient Air*. For which End the great *Canisters* are necessary for a large Quantity, and the *Tottaneg*, or *Pewter*, or *Tin Pots* for a small, whether it be sent into the Countrey, or design'd to be kept at home; and none of it should be 'er expos'd as little as may be, from such a Cover. But yet 'tis observ'd that those that endeavour to preserve the *Spirit* and *Nature* of it longest, and with least Damage, dispose of it commonly in large Tubs, which contain many Pounds, by the Bulk of which the strength of it is encreas'd against all harmful Impressions from *without*, and the Virtue of it is maintain'd more intirely within. And hence it is, that as in *Wine*, so in *Tea*, the choicest commonly is in the Middle; and that *Canister* whose

out-

ure and Qualities of T E A.

...de *Tea* may prove but ordi-
..., as being nearest the Air
... Danger, may yet upon a
...er search be found to con-
... what is far more valuable.
... *Age*, *Air*, and *Damp*, inevita-
... destroy those Sorts of *Tea*,
...ch is quite out of its Ele-
...t either in a moist or an
... place

Having thus far discours'd of
... *various Kinds* of this foreign
..., and the *Season* wherein it
...ld be gather'd, of the *Me-*
d of making choice of the best,
... the *Means* whereby it is *pre-*
...'d; the Reader now will ex-
...t to here something of its
...alifications, and what the *Vir-*
...s of it are, that have rais'd it
... this general eminent Esteem.
...d if we may believe those
...rsons who have been most con-
...rsant with this healthful Liquor,

The Qualities of Tea.

An ESSAY upon the [...]

quor, and receiv'd it so long [...]
the Nature of their comm[on]
Drink, we must needs enter[tain]
some Esteem for its Excellen[ce,]
and harbour a valuable Opin[ion]
of it. For the *Gout* and *St[one,]*
those painful Diseases which [so]
frequently torment the *Europea[ns,]*
are scarce known in *China,* [and]
among those most *Eastern A[sia-]*
ticks, the Happiness of whi[ch]
they commonly ascribe to t[he]
constant Use of this Liquor [a-]
mong them. The Priviledge [...]
which they reckon upon as a sp[e-]
cial Blessing to those Nation[s,]
especially when attended w[ith]
such remarkable Effects. And [as]
the intolerable Pains of these D[is-]
tempers are caus'd by an *acri[-]*
monious Juice, and some *ferme[nt]*
that is *sowre*, this Liquor is sai[d]
to mitigate the *Salt*, disturb th[e]
Tartar, and dissolve its *gravel[ly]*
Particles. When 'tis much and of[ten]

Marg: [note]
[...] the Gout
and Stone.

ture and Qualities of TEA.

drunk. For since it is an
...d that coagulates the *Blood*,
...afterwards precipitates the
...ser Parts of it into *Gravel*;
...Liquor, as some imagin,
...htily corrects the *Acid*, and
...vents the *Precipitation*. And
...ugh the Seeds of these Disea-
..., if they are *Hereditary* or
...onical, cannot easily be re-
...v'd, yet may they in some
...asure, by a daily Use of this
...ellent Drink, be much *dimi-*
...'d, or at least be kept from
...*Increase*; Especially if it be
...nk in such a *Quantity*, and
...such convenient *Times*, when
...Stomach is rather empty than
...er charg'd. For then is a Pas-
...e easily made, and with greater
...eedom both to the *Veins*, and
...the *Reins*. For a Medicine so
...ry weak and light as this, can-
...t readily conquer those Ob-
...uctions that oppose it, nor
make

make its way through them
Facility. And several Exam[ples]
might be produc'd, I que[stion]
not, among our selves, to [con]firm
the Subserviency of [this]
Leaf to these great and [useful]
Ends.

A Help to Digestion.

Nor are the *Tartars*, who [are]
now Masters of this large [and]
flourishing Empire of *China*,
sensible of the Benefit of this [In]fusion,
or Strangers to the [Vir]tue
and *Usefulness* of it.
whereas these persons are by [Na]ture
very hardy, and have so [far]
improv'd this hardiness by [Cu]stom,
that *raw Horse-flesh* is th[eir]
ordinary Food; and this they [eat]
and digest with the same F[aci]lity,
as we do Beef that's bo[il'd]
or roasted. Now hereupon h[ow]ever
it sometimes happens t[hat]
their Stomachs are oppress'd w[ith]
Crudities, and mightily weake[n'd]
throu[gh]

ough *Indigestion*; to cure
ich, they readily apply them-
es to *Tea*, without consulting
y other Physick; and in this
y find so much Relief, and
ir Appetites are so effectually
engthen'd, that they soon re-
er their Digestive Faculty a-
n and remove the *languid In-
position*. But the Leaf which
most powerful upon this occa-
is very harsh, course and
pleasant, and only grows in
Northern Province of *Xensi*,
st of which lies between 35
40 deg. of Latitude. Which
ur'eress renders it far more a-
eable to the strong Constitu-
n of the stout and robust *Tar-
than to that of the delicate
soft *Chinese*. And that this
a Virtue very remarkable in
, it seems from hence very
bable, in that the Liquor im-
gnated with its Particles will

soften

soften Flesh, *Le Compte*, p. 2
and renders hard Meats tende
whereby we may judge that
haftens *Diffolution*, and thereup
facilitates *Digestion*. Besides,
soft pointed Volatile *Salt* whe
with it abounds, and the *hot*
ter wherein it is infus'd, do mig
tily repair the natural *Fluidity*
the *Juices* of the Body, and
a gentle Aftriction agreeably f
tify the Tone of the *Bowels*, a
of a weak *Stomach*; vide *Pec*
de Po *Ilex Dialogum*, p.
And if this therefore be a Q
lity inherent in this Liquor,
ftrengthen a taint Appetite, a
correct the naufeous Humours t
offend the Stomach, it muft nee
in fome meafure happily cont
bute to the Health of fome we
and feeble Conftitutions, and li
wife throw off abundance of th
Crudities created in the Bo
through *Excess*. And by t
mea

ature and Qualities of TEA.

[...]eans, that the Vigour of the Ap-
[...]tite is regain'd, the Sweetness
[...] the Blood may be preserv'd,
[...]d the sharpness that is in it be
[...]ated, whereby this *China* Drink
[...]ay prove a friendly Remedy a-
[...]inst the *Scurvy*, that Northern
[...]pular Disease, and become as
[...]uable a Blessing to us, as it
[...] the *Tartars*, who fall in-
[...] same Distemper with us,
[...]n the very same Account, of
[...] gross and high Feeding.

A Remedy for the Scurvy.

The last Remark which I shall
[...]ake of this innocent lovely Li-
[...]or, is the Advantage which it
[...]s over *Wine*, and the Ascen-
[...]nt which it gains over the pow-
[...]ful Juice of the Grape, which
[...] frequently betrays Men into
[...] much Mischief, and so many
[...]ollies. For this Admirable *Tea*
[...]deavours to reconcile Men to
[...]*briety*, when their Brains are

It prevails over the Fumes of Wine.

over-

overcast with the Fumes of In-
temperance, and disorder'd wi[th]
Excess of Drinking, by driv[ing]
away the superfluous Humors th[at]
cloud the Rational Faculty, a[nd]
disturb the Powers of the Mi[nd].
And therefore all those Perso[ns]
who have by this means lost th[eir]
Senses, and have past the Boun[ds]
of Moderation, ought presen[tly]
to water their Veins with t[his Li]-
quor, and refresh themselves w[ith]
its sober Draughts, if they a[re]
willing to recollect their rov[ing]
Thoughts, and be Masters [of]
their Faculties again. For th[ere]
is none of its meanest Triumph[s]
that 'tis able to subdue this co[n]-
quering Liquor, that has fo[iled]
so many wise and powerful, th[at]
it is an *Anti Circe*, can counte[r]
charm the inchanted Cup, a[nd]
change the Beast into a Ma[n].

*Vertiginem capitisque dolorem (p[rae]-
sertim à crapula ortum) mitig[at]*

...p. 15. And that it is
...altogether destitute of this
...markable Faculty of suppressing
...ours in the Brain, seems not
...probable from what is observed
...it in *China*. For when any
...e there is unfortunately seiz'd vertigo
...'a *Vertigo*, through a Redun-
...nce of Humours towards the
...ead, the Use of this Liquor is
...en a kind Relief to this Di-
...mper by obstructing the Paf-
...ge of the Steam from the Sto-
...ach and lower Parts. Because
...e thick Vapours that continually
...end, being the Cause of this
...sturbance, whenever they are
...eck'd and controll'd in their
...iage by the lively Spirit
...f. the *Megrim* sensibly a-
...tes. For *Tea* has none of that
...ry Spirit that inflames the
...ood and disorders the Chan-
...sins of the Brain, and is the pro-
...er Vice of *Wine*; 'tis quick in

deed and active is that Liqu[or,]
but happily destitute of all [an]
intoxicating Quality. It ne[ver]
ascends into the Brain, but th[at]
'tis with a Candid Design of [pu]rifying and of quickening it, [not]
immediately to render it mudd[y,]
sluggish and confus'd. And up[on]
this score it justly claims an [in]terest and Share in the A[cti]ons of all Men of fanciful a[nd]
sprightly Thoughts, of all th[at]
would Animate their Facult[ies]
without Disturbance, and ma[in]tain their Idea lively and brig[ht,]
in that it actuates and quicke[ns]
the drowsy Thoughts, adds a ki[nd]
of new Soul to the *Fancy*, a[nd]
gives fresh Vigour and Force [to]
the wearied *Invention*. As so[me]
ingenious Persons in th[is] Kingdo[m]
by frequent Experience can tes[ti]fy.

...ature and Qualities of TEA.

And if Ingenuity may be al-
...'d to have a Vote here, I
... produce that which is unque-
...nable in the Testimony of
... Hales, whose Character of
... Herb may be seen in these
...ses.

... TEA, commended by
Her MAJESTY.

Venus her Myrtle, Phœbus has
  his Bays,
...A both excels, which she vouch-
...afes to praise.
...best of Queens, and best of Herbs
...we...
...old Nation, which the way
...d show
...e fair Region, where the Sun
...es rise;

Whose rich Productions we so justly
    prize.
The Muses friend, TEA, does our
    Fancy aid;
Repress those Vapors which the Head
    invade:
And keeps that Palace of the Soul se-
    rene,
Fit on her Birth Day to Salute the
    Queen.

And keep Men waking

And from this Eminent Property which it has of animating the Faculties, and keeping up the Vigor of the Spirits, arises that other remarkable Power which it gains over *Sleep* and *Drowsiness*, and the natural Inclination of the Body to Rest. So that a few Cups of this Excellent Liquor will soon rowze the cloudy Vapours that benight the Brain, and drive away all Mists from the Eyes. 'Tis a kind of another *Phœbus* to the Soul, both for its
    Spirit

…*ature and Qualities of* TEA. 33

…*ring* and *inlightning* it; and
…spight of all the Darkness of
…Night, and all the Heaviness
…the Mind, 'twill brighten and
…mate the Thoughts, and expel
…ose Mists of Humours that
…ll and darken Meditation. Ac-
…ding to Dr. *Chamberlain's* Ac-
…unt in his Treatise of *Tea*;
…*en I have been*, says he, *com-*
…l'd to sit up all Night about some
…traordinary Business, I needed to
…no more than to take some of
…s Tea, when I perceiv'd my self
…inning to sleep, and I could easily
…tch all Night without winking;
…l in the Morning I was as
…sh as if I had slept my ordinary
…e; this I could do once a Week
…hout any trouble. And this
…tainly must gain it a mighty
…neration from all those Sons of
…*Muses*, who labour in the
…ght, and are desirous to keep
…ir *Memories* fresh, and their

C 4 *Sen-*

Senses waking; and endeavo[ur]
to prolong those Hours that [are]
devoted to studious Thoughts, [the]
Strength and Clearness of Und[er]
standing; Because at such tim[es]
in the Use of this sprightly [Li]
quor, they perceive a speedy [Re]
medy against their natural W[ea]
riness and Stupidity.

And that the several Virt[ues]
which are here ascrib'd to t[his]
delicate Leaf or not meerly N[o]
tional, or of bare conjecture, [the]
Testimonies of several emin[ent]
Authors might be produced, [such]
as *Ray's* Histor. Plant. *Olaus* W[or]
mius in Musæo, p. 165. *Tulp*
Observat l. 4. cap. ult &c. [But]
the Account of one of them o[nly]
shall be at present sufficient. T[he]
Learned *Michael Etmuller*, P[ro]
fessor of Physick at *Lypsick*, [in]
the third Edition of his Notes [on]
Schroder's Pharmacy, publish[ed]

Nature and Qualities of TEA.

by his Scholar Dr. *John Caspar* of *Westphalia*, gives an Account of the Herb *Tcha*, or *Tea*, to this purpose; *It powerfully Corrects Indigestions and Crudities, so as that the very* Chinese *use this Drink to strengthen the first Digestion, and to purify the Mass of Blood by a Flux of Urine. Whence it is that they rarely labour under the Hypocondriack Passion, descended from a deprav'd Stomach: For* Tcha's *Aromatick Virtue takes away all acid Crudities. Besides, it is a very famous Cephalick, adds a wonderful Strength to the Animal Spirits, and by that means opposes the Megrim, and admirably comforts the Memory, and other Faculties of the Soul. Moreover, it drives away Drowsiness, and keeps a Man awake without Weariness.*

It is a most noble Antinephritick and Antipodagick; Whereupon they

that

that take this Drink, are not subject to the Stone and Gravel, while it partly *drives it out, and partly destroys the praeternatural Acid in the Stomach and Guts, and likewise in the Blood, (volatilizing it, if coagulated by an Acid) in which Respect it preserves both from the Stone and Gout, whereby the Chinese and Japanese are rarely, if ever, infested with them.* All which admirable Effects, and much more, are confirm'd by the most famous *Wilhelmus ten Rhine*, Physician, Botanist, and Chymist to the Emperor of *Japan*, in his Discourse *De Frutice Thee*; who there affirms too, that *it both prevails against the Dropsy, and is an Antidote extraordinary against the Weakness of the Sight.*

But notwithstanding all this Authority, this Leaf has formerly been Subject to Reproach and Ca-

…ature and *Qualities of T E A.*

…vil. And it were a happy
…af indeed were it altogether
…bjection-free, and out of the
…each of Enmity and Contra-
…ction. But however, this Hap-
…ness it has That herein it shares
…te with all things that are ex-
…llent, which are often aspers'd
… for their *Innocence,* and in *Two Objections*
… respect owe all their Mi- *answer'd.*
…ry to their Perfection. That
…hich was wont to be argued
… Disparagement of that general
…redit which this Drink by its
…erits has obtained, was, That
… was a Parent to the *Cholick* and
…*abates,* though it was very use-
…l upon other Accounts; and that
… unhappily caus'd these Diseases
…nong us. But notwithstanding
…at 'tis very well known, that
…ese are no upstart Distempers
…re, but challenge a Standing
… ancient Date; yet were they
…e necessary Consequence of the
Use

An ESSAY upon the Use of this Modern Liquor [in] England, all the Eastern Nations, especially China, India, and [Japan], must needs be sorely afflicted with them; and therefore [a great] deal of encouraging as they [must] rather renounce their [beloved] Drink unless they a[re] [ever pleas]'d with it, [along] with their Health. And yet w[e] never [hear] that these Dis[eases] are complain'd of there, though [this] Liquor is as familiarly us[ed by] them, as Small Beer is w[ith] us; and that not only by th[e] Natives, but by several Europ[ean]s, who are nevertheless alto[gether] Strangers to the Painfulne[ss] of those Maladies. If the D[ist]e[mp]er derives it self from this Fou[n]tain, how comes it to pass th[at] that among all the numerous A[dmi]rers of Tea, so very few labo[ur] under that Distemper? And as t[o] the Cholick, many Skilful Pract[i]tione[rs]

Nature and Qualities of TEA.

tioners in Physick do observe, that several Persons of Interior Note in *England*, whose Fortune never rais'd them to the Character of being *Tea drinkers*, are more disturb'd with that Distemper, than such as plentifully drink it daily.

Yet some will urge, That although these Virtues which I have mention'd may be fairly attributed to this *China* Liquor, yet are they sometimes obstructed by the use of that Sugar which is commonly mix'd with it. And this indeed, I must confess, may somewhat abate the Efficacy of it in some Operations; yet this Advantage it produces, in benefitting of the *Lungs* and *Reins*; to which it is a mighty Friend.

And yet after all, though these rare and excellent Qualities have long been observeable in *Tea*, yet must

must we not imagine that they always meet with the same Effect indifferently in all Persons, or that they universally prevail. For either the *Height* of a Distemper, or the long *Continuance* of it, either the *Constitution* of the Person, or some certain *occult Indisposition* may avert the Efficacy and Obstruct or delay the desired Success. It may either be drunk without *Advice*, or at *unseasonable Times*; either the *Water* or the *Tea*, may be bad; and if the *Flask* it self be sickly, we cannot easily expect much *Health* by it.

FINIS.

Milton Keynes UK
Ingram Content Group UK Ltd.
UKHW050709051224
3433UKWH00048B/648